OSTEOARTHRITIS DIET COOKBOOK

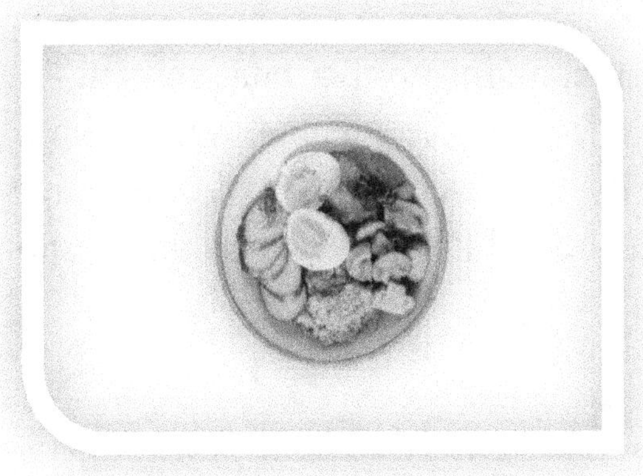

The complete osteoarthritis nutrition guide with delicious and nutritious anti-inflammatory recipes for joint pain relief

Dr. Mary D. Cook

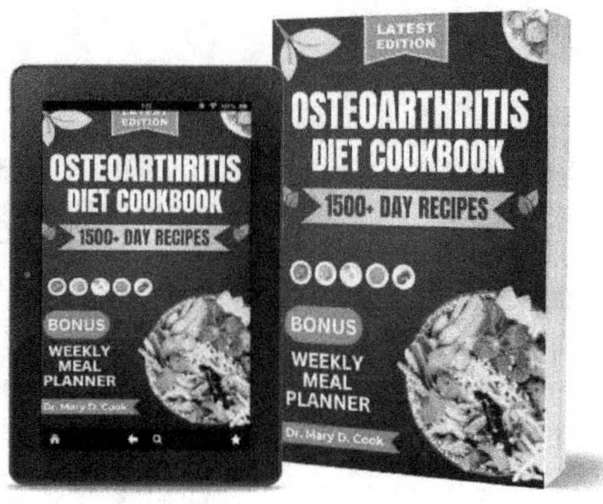
LATEST EDITION
OSTEOARTHRITIS
DIET COOKBOOK
1500+ DAY RECIPES
BONUS
WEEKLY MEAL PLANNER
Dr. Mary D. Cook
LATEST EDITION
OSTEOARTHRITIS
DIET COOKBOOK
1500+ DAY RECIPES
BONUS
WEEKLY MEAL PLANNER
Dr. Mary D. Cook

TABLE OF CONTENTS

OTHER BOOKS BY THE AUTHOR

1. OSTEOPOROSIS DIET COOKBOOK FOR SENIORS

CLICK HERE TO GET YOUR COPY NOW!!!

2. THE ULTIMATE OSTEOPOROSIS DIET COOKBOOK FOR WOMEN

CLICK HERE TO GET YOUR COPY NOW!!!

3. THE ULTIMATE GASTRIC SLEEVE BARIATRIC COOKBOOK

CLICK HERE TO GET YOUR COPY!!!

4. PESCATARIAN DIET COOKBOOK FOR DIABETICS

CLICK HER TO GET YOUR COPY NOW!!!

5. MEDITERRANEAN DIET COOKBOOK FOR RHEUMATOID ARTHRITIS

CLICK HERE TO GET YOUR COPY NOW!!!

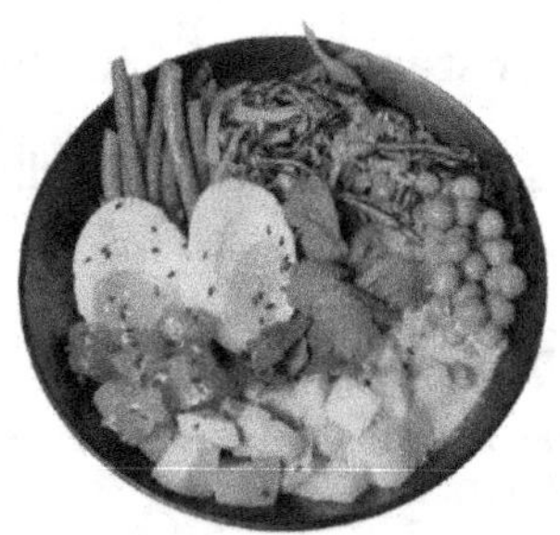

INTRODUCTION

Welcome to the "OSTEOARTHRITIS DIET COOKBOOK: The complete osteoarthritis nutrition guide with delicious and nutritious anti-inflammatory recipes for joint pain relief." I'm thrilled to embark on this journey with you, sharing my passion for nutrition and offering valuable insights into how dietary choices can profoundly impact our health, particularly for those grappling with osteoarthritis.

Allow me to introduce myself. I'm **Dr. Mary D. Cook**, a dedicated nutritionist with a wealth of experience spanning several years. My journey into the realm of nutrition wasn't merely a career choice; it was a deeply personal odyssey fueled by a desire to understand and harness the transformative power of food to heal and nourish the body.

My own battle with osteoarthritis ignited a fervent quest for knowledge, leading me down avenues of research, experimentation, and ultimately, profound revelation. Like many of you, I once found myself ensnared in the grip of joint pain, grappling with the limitations it imposed on my daily life. Yet, within that struggle lay the seeds of resilience and determination that would ultimately shape my path towards healing.

The turning point came when I began to recognize the pivotal role that nutrition plays in mitigating inflammation, bolstering joint health, and alleviating the symptoms of osteoarthritis. Armed with this newfound understanding, I embarked on a transformative journey that would not only restore vitality to my own life but would also ignite a fervent commitment to empowering others on their own paths towards wellness.

Through meticulous research, hands-on experimentation, and a deep reverence for the healing power of nature's bounty, I honed a repertoire of recipes designed specifically to combat inflammation, soothe joint pain, and nurture overall well-being. The recipes contained within this cookbook are not merely culinary creations; they are the culmination of years of dedication, informed by the latest scientific insights and infused with a passion for wholesome, flavorful cuisine.

But perhaps what resonates most deeply within these pages is the recognition that the journey towards healing is not merely a solitary endeavor—it is a collective pursuit fueled by shared knowledge, support, and encouragement.

As you embark on this culinary adventure, I invite you to embrace the potential for transformation that lies within each recipe, each ingredient, and each nourishing meal.

In these pages, you'll find a treasure trove of delectable dishes crafted with care and intention, each one carefully curated to deliver not only exquisite flavors but also potent anti-inflammatory benefits. From vibrant salads bursting with fresh produce to hearty stews brimming with wholesome ingredients, each recipe is a testament to the remarkable synergy between nutrition and wellness.

But beyond the realm of culinary delights lies a profound truth: that healing begins with a single step, a single choice, a single bite. As you embark on this journey, know that you are not alone. Together, we can harness the power of nutrition to unlock the door to vitality, resilience, and enduring well-being.

So, let us embark on this journey together, guided by the shared vision of a future where vibrant health and vitality are within reach for all. Welcome to the "OSTEOARTHRITIS DIET COOKBOOK," where delicious flavors, nourishing ingredients, and the transformative power of nutrition converge to pave the way towards a life lived to the fullest.

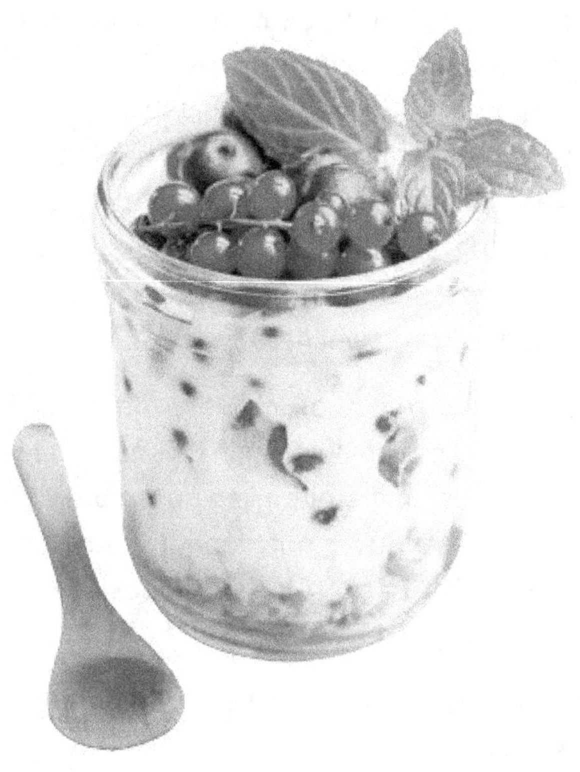

PART 1:

Osteoarthritis (OA) is the most common form of arthritis, affecting millions of people worldwide. It is a chronic degenerative joint disease characterized by the breakdown of cartilage in the joints, leading to pain, stiffness, and reduced mobility. Understanding the nature of osteoarthritis, its types, causes, symptoms, and preventive measures is crucial for managing the condition effectively and improving quality of life.

Understanding Osteoarthritis:

Osteoarthritis primarily affects the joints, where the protective cartilage that cushions the ends of bones wears down over time. Without this cushioning, the bones may rub against each other, leading to pain, inflammation, and eventual joint damage. While osteoarthritis can occur in any joint, it most commonly affects the knees, hips, hands, and spine.

Types of Osteoarthritis:

There are two main types of osteoarthritis:

1. Primary Osteoarthritis: This type of osteoarthritis occurs due to the natural aging process and wear and tear on the joints over time.

Factors such as genetics, joint injuries, obesity, and repetitive stress on the joints can contribute to the development of primary osteoarthritis.

2. Secondary Osteoarthritis: Secondary osteoarthritis develops as a result of an underlying condition or injury that affects joint health. Examples include joint injuries, obesity, metabolic disorders, congenital joint abnormalities, and inflammatory joint diseases like rheumatoid arthritis.

Causes of Osteoarthritis:

Several factors can contribute to the development of osteoarthritis:

1. **Age:** Osteoarthritis is more common in older adults, as the natural wear and tear on the joints over time can lead to cartilage breakdown.

2. **Obesity:** Excess weight puts added stress on weight-bearing joints such as the knees and hips, increasing the risk of osteoarthritis.

3. **Joint Injuries:** Previous joint injuries, such as fractures or ligament tears, can predispose individuals to osteoarthritis later in life.

4. **Genetics:** Family history plays a role in the development of osteoarthritis, suggesting a genetic predisposition to the condition.

5. **Joint Overuse:** Repetitive stress on the joints due to certain occupations, sports activities, or manual labor can contribute to the development of osteoarthritis.

6. **Other Health Conditions:** Certain metabolic disorders, inflammatory joint diseases, and congenital joint abnormalities can increase the risk of osteoarthritis.

Symptoms of Osteoarthritis:

The symptoms of osteoarthritis can vary depending on the severity of the condition and the joints affected. **Common symptoms include:**

1. **Joint Pain:** Pain and discomfort in the affected joints, particularly during movement or weight-bearing activities.

2. **Stiffness:** Joint stiffness, especially after periods of inactivity or upon waking in the morning.

3. **Swelling:** Swelling and inflammation around the affected joints, often accompanied by warmth and tenderness to the touch.

4. **Decreased Range of Motion:** Difficulty moving the affected joint through its full range of motion, leading to stiffness and reduced flexibility.

5. **Joint Instability:** Feeling of joint instability or weakness, particularly in weight-bearing joints like the knees and hips.

6. **Bone Spurs:** Formation of bone spurs (osteophytes) around the edges of the affected joints, which can contribute to joint pain and inflammation.

7. **Joint Deformities:** In advanced cases, osteoarthritis can lead to joint deformities and loss of function.

Preventive Measures for Osteoarthritis:

While certain risk factors for osteoarthritis, such as age and genetics, cannot be modified, there are several preventive measures individuals can take to reduce their risk of developing the condition or manage its progression:

1. **Maintain a Healthy Weight:** Maintaining a healthy weight reduces the stress on weight-bearing joints, such as the knees and hips, lowering the risk of osteoarthritis and alleviating symptoms in those already affected.

2. **Stay Active:** Regular exercise helps strengthen the muscles around the joints, improve joint flexibility, and maintain overall joint health.

Low-impact activities such as walking, swimming, and cycling are particularly beneficial for individuals with osteoarthritis.

3. **Avoid Joint Overuse:** Avoid repetitive stress on the joints by practicing proper body mechanics, taking regular breaks during repetitive tasks, and using ergonomic tools and equipment when necessary.

4. **Protect Your Joints:** Wear supportive footwear, use joint braces or splints as needed, and avoid activities that put excessive strain on the joints.

5. **Adopt a Healthy Diet:** A balanced diet rich in fruits, vegetables, whole grains, lean proteins, and healthy fats can help reduce inflammation, support joint health, and promote overall well-being.

6. **Manage Stress:** Chronic stress can exacerbate inflammation and contribute to joint pain. Practice stress-reduction techniques such as mindfulness meditation, deep breathing exercises, or yoga to promote relaxation and alleviate tension.

7. **Stay Hydrated:** Drinking an adequate amount of water helps keep the joints lubricated and supports overall joint health.

8. **Quit Smoking:** Smoking has been linked to an increased risk of osteoarthritis and can worsen symptoms in those already affected. Quitting smoking can help reduce inflammation and improve overall joint health.

9. **Get Regular Check-ups:** Regular medical check-ups allow for early detection and management of underlying health conditions that may increase the risk of osteoarthritis.

10. **Follow Treatment Recommendations:** If diagnosed with osteoarthritis, work closely with healthcare professionals to develop a personalized treatment plan that may include medications, physical therapy, lifestyle modifications, and other interventions to manage symptoms and slow disease progression.

Understanding the types, causes, symptoms, and preventive measures of osteoarthritis is essential for effectively managing the condition and improving quality of life. By adopting healthy lifestyle habits, staying active, and seeking appropriate medical care, you can reduce your risk of developing osteoarthritis and effectively manage its symptoms to maintain overall joint health and well-being.

PART 2:

Achieving optimum health while managing osteoarthritis involves adopting a balanced diet rich in nutrients that support joint health, reduce inflammation, and promote overall well-being. By incorporating specific foods and avoiding others, individuals can optimize their nutrition to alleviate symptoms, slow disease progression, and enhance quality of life.

Foods to Eat:

1. **Omega-3 Fatty Acids:** Omega-3 fatty acids found in fatty fish such as salmon, mackerel, and sardines have anti-inflammatory properties that can help reduce joint pain and inflammation associated with osteoarthritis.

2. **Fruits and Vegetables:** Colorful fruits and vegetables are rich in antioxidants and phytonutrients that help combat inflammation and support overall joint health. Aim to include a variety of fruits and vegetables in your diet, such as berries, oranges, leafy greens, broccoli, and bell peppers.

3. **Whole Grains:** Whole grains like brown rice, quinoa, oats, and whole wheat are high in fiber and nutrients that help maintain stable blood sugar levels and reduce inflammation.

4. **Nuts and Seeds:** Nuts and seeds such as walnuts, almonds, flaxseeds, and chia seeds are rich in omega-3 fatty acids, antioxidants, and other nutrients that support joint health and reduce inflammation.

5. **Healthy Fats:** Incorporate sources of healthy fats such as olive oil, avocados, and coconut oil into your diet. These fats have anti-inflammatory properties and can help reduce joint pain and stiffness.

6. **Lean Protein:** Choose lean sources of protein such as poultry, fish, tofu, legumes, and beans. Protein is essential for muscle repair and maintenance, which is important for supporting joint health and mobility.

7. **Low-fat Dairy:** Low-fat dairy products like yogurt and milk provide calcium and vitamin D, which are important for maintaining strong bones and overall joint health.

8. **Herbs and Spices:** Incorporate herbs and spices such as turmeric, ginger, cinnamon, and garlic into your cooking. These spices have anti-inflammatory properties and can help reduce joint pain and inflammation.

Foods to Avoid:

1. **Processed Foods:** Processed foods like sugary snacks, fast food, and pre-packaged meals often contain high levels of unhealthy fats, sugar, and sodium, which can exacerbate inflammation and contribute to joint pain.

2. **Saturated and Trans Fats:** Limit your intake of saturated and trans fats found in fried foods, red meat, processed meats, and full-fat dairy products. These fats can promote inflammation and increase the risk of heart disease.

3. **Refined Carbohydrates:** Foods made with refined grains such as white bread, white rice, and sugary cereals should be limited. These foods can cause spikes in blood sugar levels and promote inflammation.

4. **Excessive Alcohol:** Limit your intake of alcohol, as excessive consumption can increase inflammation and worsen joint pain. Stick to moderate amounts of alcohol, if any, and choose healthier alternatives like water, herbal tea, or infused water.

5. **Added Sugars:** Minimize your consumption of foods and beverages high in added sugars, such as soda, candy, and baked goods. These sugary treats can contribute to inflammation and joint pain.

6. **High-Sodium Foods:** Reduce your intake of high-sodium foods like processed meats, canned soups, and salty snacks. Excess sodium can lead to water retention and inflammation, exacerbating joint symptoms.

7. **Nightshade Vegetables (for Some):** Some individuals with osteoarthritis may find that nightshade vegetables such as tomatoes, peppers, eggplants, and potatoes worsen their symptoms. Pay attention to your body's response to these foods and consider eliminating or reducing them if they exacerbate joint pain or inflammation.

In conclusion, achieving optimum health on an osteoarthritis diet involves focusing on nutrient-dense foods that support joint health, reduce inflammation, and promote overall well-being. By incorporating omega-3 fatty acids, fruits, vegetables, whole grains, nuts, seeds, lean protein, healthy fats, and herbs/spices into your diet while limiting processed foods, unhealthy fats, refined carbohydrates, alcohol, added sugars, high-sodium foods, and potentially problematic nightshade vegetables, you can optimize your nutrition to alleviate symptoms and improve quality of life. Additionally, staying hydrated, maintaining a healthy weight, and practicing portion control are important aspects of a balanced osteoarthritis diet.

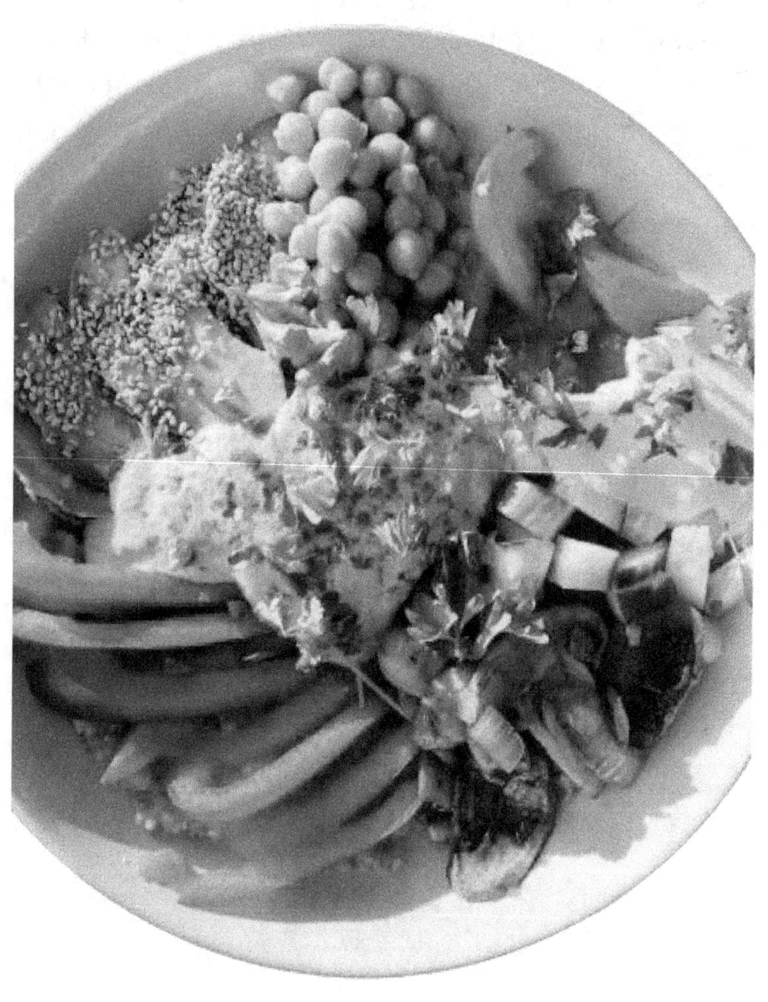

PART 3:

Delicious osteoarthritis-friendly breakfast recipes:

1. Avocado and Spinach Omelette

Ingredients:

- 2 eggs, 1/4 avocado, sliced
- 1/2 cup fresh spinach leaves
- Salt and pepper to taste
- 1 tsp olive oil

Instructions:

1. In a bowl, whisk the eggs with salt and pepper.
2. Heat olive oil in a non-stick skillet over medium heat.
3. Pour the egg mixture into the skillet and tilt to spread evenly.
4. Once the edges begin to set, add the avocado slices and spinach on one side of the omelette.
5. Fold the other side of the omelette over the filling and cook for another minute.

6. Slide the omelette onto a plate, slice, and serve hot.

Servings: 1 **Nutritional Value (per serving):** Calories: 250, Protein: 14g, Fat: 18g, Carbohydrates: 6g **Cooking Time:** 10 minutes

2. Greek Yogurt Parfait

Ingredients:

- 1/2 cup Greek yogurt

- 1/4 cup mixed berries (such as strawberries, blueberries, raspberries)

- 1 tbsp chopped almonds or walnuts

- 1 tsp honey (optional)

Instructions:

1. In a glass or bowl, layer Greek yogurt, mixed berries, and chopped nuts.

2. Drizzle with honey if desired.

3. Repeat layers if desired.

4. Serve immediately.

Servings: 1 **Nutritional Value (per serving):** Calories: 200, Protein: 15g, Fat: 8g, Carbohydrates: 20g **Cooking Time:** 5 minutes

Ingredients:

- 1 whole wheat tortilla
- 2 eggs, scrambled
- 1/4 cup sliced mushrooms
- 1/2 cup fresh spinach leaves
- Salt and pepper to taste
- 1 tsp olive oil

Instructions:

1. Heat olive oil in a skillet over medium heat.
2. Add sliced mushrooms and cook until softened.
3. Add fresh spinach leaves and cook until wilted.
4. Season scrambled eggs with salt and pepper, then add them to the skillet.
5. Cook, stirring gently, until the eggs are set.
6. Place the egg, mushroom, and spinach mixture in the center of the whole wheat tortilla.
7. Fold in the sides of the tortilla and roll up tightly.
8. Cut the wrap in half and serve warm.

Servings: 1 **Nutritional Value (per serving):** Calories: 300, Protein: 20g, Fat: 12g, Carbohydrates: 25g **Cooking Time:** 15 minutes

4. Overnight Chia Seed Pudding

Ingredients:

- 2 tbsp chia seeds

- 1/2 cup unsweetened almond milk

- 1/4 tsp vanilla extract

- 1/2 cup mixed berries

- 1 tbsp chopped almonds or walnuts

Instructions:

1. In a bowl or jar, mix chia seeds, almond milk, and vanilla extract.

2. Stir well to combine and ensure there are no clumps.

3. Cover and refrigerate overnight or for at least 4 hours.

4. In the morning, stir the chia seed pudding and top with mixed berries and chopped nuts.

5. Serve chilled.

Servings: 1 **Nutritional Value (per serving):** Calories: 250, Protein: 8g, Fat: 15g, Carbohydrates: 20g **Preparation Time:** 5 minutes (plus refrigeration time)

5. Quinoa Breakfast Bowl

Ingredients:

- 1/2 cup cooked quinoa

- 1/4 cup Greek yogurt

- 1/4 cup mixed berries

- 1 tbsp chopped almonds or walnuts

- 1 tsp honey (optional)

Instructions:

1. In a bowl, layer cooked quinoa, Greek yogurt, mixed berries, and chopped nuts.

2. Drizzle with honey if desired.

3. Serve immediately.

Servings: 1 **Nutritional Value (per serving):** Calories: 300, Protein: 15g, Fat: 8g, Carbohydrates: 35g **Cooking Time:** 15 minutes (for cooking quinoa)

Ingredients:

- 4 eggs
- 1/4 cup diced bell peppers
- 1/4 cup diced onions
- 1/4 cup diced tomatoes
- 1/4 cup chopped spinach
- Salt and pepper to taste
- 1/4 cup shredded low-fat cheese (optional)

Instructions:

1. Preheat the oven to 350°F (175°C).
2. In a bowl, whisk the eggs with salt and pepper.
3. Stir in diced bell peppers, onions, tomatoes, and chopped spinach.
4. Pour the mixture into a greased baking dish.
5. Bake for 20-25 minutes or until the eggs are set.
6. Sprinkle shredded cheese on top if desired and bake for an additional 5 minutes until melted.
7. Slice into squares and serve hot.

Servings: 2 **Nutritional Value (per serving):** Calories: 200, Protein: 12g, Fat: 10g, Carbohydrates: 15g **Cooking Time:** 30 minutes

7. Banana and Almond Butter Toast

Ingredients:

- 1 slice whole wheat bread, toasted

- 1 tbsp almond butter

- 1/2 banana, sliced

- Cinnamon for sprinkling (optional)

Instructions:

1. Spread almond butter evenly on the toasted whole wheat bread.

2. Top with sliced bananas.

3. Sprinkle with cinnamon if desired.

4. Serve immediately.

Servings: 1 **Nutritional Value (per serving):** Calories: 250, Protein: 7g, Fat: 12g, Carbohydrates: 30g **Cooking Time:** 5 minutes

Ingredients:

- 1/2 cup frozen mixed berries
- 1/2 cup fresh spinach leaves
- 1/2 cup unsweetened almond milk
- 1/4 cup Greek yogurt
- 1 tbsp chia seeds

Instructions:

1. Place all ingredients in a blender.
2. Blend until smooth and creamy.
3. Pour into a glass and serve immediately.

Servings: 1 **Nutritional Value (per serving):** Calories: 200, Protein: 10g, Fat: 8g, Carbohydrates: 25g

Preparation Time: 5 minutes

Ingredients:

- 1 small sweet potato, peeled and diced
- 1/4 cup diced bell peppers
- 1/4 cup diced onions
- 1/4 cup diced tomatoes
- 1/4 cup chopped spinach
- Salt and pepper to taste
- 1 tsp olive oil
- 2 eggs

Instructions:

1. Heat olive oil in a skillet over medium heat.
2. Add diced sweet potatoes and cook until tender.
3. Add diced bell peppers, onions, tomatoes, and chopped spinach.
4. Season with salt and pepper and cook until vegetables are softened.
5. Push the vegetables to one side of the skillet and crack the eggs into the other side.

6. Cook the eggs until desired doneness.

7. Serve the sweet potato hash topped with fried eggs.

Servings: 2 **Nutritional Value (per serving):** Calories: 250, Protein: 12g, Fat: 10g, Carbohydrates: 25g **Cooking Time:** 20 minutes

10. Almond Flour Pancakes

Ingredients:

- 1/2 cup almond flour

- 2 eggs

- 1/4 cup unsweetened almond milk

- 1/2 tsp baking powder

- 1/4 tsp vanilla extract

- Pinch of salt

- 1 tsp olive oil (for cooking)

Instructions:

1. In a bowl, whisk together almond flour, eggs, almond milk, baking powder, vanilla extract, and salt until smooth.

2. Heat olive oil in a skillet over medium heat.

3. Pour the pancake batter onto the skillet to form small pancakes.

4. Cook for 2-3 minutes on each side or until golden brown.

5. Serve hot with your favorite toppings such as fresh berries, Greek yogurt, or a drizzle of honey.

Servings: 2 (4 small pancakes each) **Nutritional Value (per serving):** Calories: 200, Protein: 10g, Fat: 15g, Carbohydrates: 10g **Cooking Time:** 10 minutes

These osteoarthritis-friendly breakfast recipes are not only delicious but also packed with nutrients to support joint health and overall well-being. Enjoy starting your day with a nutritious and satisfying meal that helps manage osteoarthritis symptoms while promoting optimal health.

Delicious osteoarthritis-friendly lunch recipes:

Ingredients:

- 2 salmon fillets

- 1 cup cooked quinoa

- 1 cup mixed vegetables (such as bell peppers, cucumber, cherry tomatoes)

- 2 tbsp olive oil

- 1 tbsp lemon juice

- Salt and pepper to taste

- Fresh herbs for garnish (such as parsley or dill)

Instructions:

1. Preheat the grill to medium-high heat.

2. Season salmon fillets with salt, pepper, and a drizzle of olive oil.

3. Grill salmon for 4-5 minutes on each side, until cooked through.

4. In a bowl, combine cooked quinoa, mixed vegetables, olive oil, lemon juice, salt, and pepper.

5. Toss to combine and adjust seasoning if needed.

6. Serve grilled salmon on a bed of quinoa salad, garnished with fresh herbs.

Servings: 2 **Nutritional Value (per serving):** Calories: 350, Protein: 25g, Fat: 18g, Carbohydrates: 20g **Cooking Time:** 20 minutes

2. Turkey and Avocado Wrap

Ingredients:

- 2 whole wheat tortillas

- 4 slices turkey breast

- 1/2 avocado, sliced

- 1/4 cup shredded lettuce

- 1/4 cup sliced bell peppers

- Mustard or hummus for spreading (optional)

Instructions:

1. Lay out the whole wheat tortillas on a clean surface.

2. Spread mustard or hummus (if using) on each tortilla.

3. Layer turkey slices, avocado slices, shredded lettuce, and sliced bell peppers on each tortilla.

4. Roll up tightly and slice in half.

5. Serve immediately or wrap in foil for later.

Servings: 2 **Nutritional Value (per serving):** Calories: 300, Protein: 20g, Fat: 12g, Carbohydrates: 25g **Preparation Time:** 10 minutes

3. Quinoa and Black Bean Stuffed Bell Peppers

Ingredients:

- 2 large bell peppers, halved and seeds removed

- 1 cup cooked quinoa

- 1/2 cup black beans, drained and rinsed

- 1/4 cup diced tomatoes

- 1/4 cup diced onions

- 1/4 cup shredded low-fat cheese (optional)

- 1 tsp olive oil

- Salt and pepper to taste

Instructions:

1. Preheat the oven to 375°F (190°C).

2. Heat olive oil in a skillet over medium heat.

3. Add diced onions and cook until softened.

4. Stir in cooked quinoa, black beans, diced tomatoes, salt, and pepper.

5. Cook for 2-3 minutes, then remove from heat.

6. Fill each bell pepper half with the quinoa and black bean mixture.

7. Place stuffed bell peppers in a baking dish and sprinkle with shredded cheese (if using).

8. Bake for 20-25 minutes or until the peppers are tender and the cheese is melted.

9. Serve hot.

Servings: 2 (1 stuffed pepper half each) **Nutritional Value (per serving):** Calories: 250, Protein: 10g, Fat: 5g, Carbohydrates: 40g **Cooking Time:** 30 minutes

Ingredients:

- 1 cup dried lentils, rinsed and drained
- 4 cups vegetable broth
- 1/2 cup diced carrots
- 1/2 cup diced celery
- 1/2 cup diced onions
- 2 cloves garlic, minced
- 1 tsp olive oil
- 1/2 tsp dried thyme
- Salt and pepper to taste
- Fresh parsley for garnish

Instructions:

1. Heat olive oil in a large pot over medium heat.
2. Add diced onions, carrots, and celery, and cook until softened.
3. Stir in minced garlic and dried thyme, and cook for another minute.
4. Add dried lentils and vegetable broth to the pot.

5. Bring to a boil, then reduce heat and simmer for 20-25 minutes or until lentils are tender.

6. Season with salt and pepper to taste.

7. Ladle soup into bowls and garnish with fresh parsley.

8. Serve hot.

Servings: 4 **Nutritional Value (per serving):** Calories: 200, Protein: 12g, Fat: 3g, Carbohydrates: 30g **Cooking Time:** 30 minutes

5. Chicken and Vegetable Stir-Fry

Ingredients:

- 2 chicken breasts, sliced

- 2 cups mixed vegetables (such as broccoli, bell peppers, snap peas)

- 2 cloves garlic, minced

- 1 tbsp soy sauce (low-sodium)

- 1 tsp sesame oil

- 1 tsp olive oil

- Cooked brown rice for serving

Instructions:

1. Heat olive oil in a large skillet or wok over medium-high heat.

2. Add sliced chicken breasts and cook until browned and cooked through.

3. Remove chicken from the skillet and set aside.

4. In the same skillet, add minced garlic and stir-fry for 30 seconds.

5. Add mixed vegetables to the skillet and stir-fry until tender-crisp.

6. Return cooked chicken to the skillet.

7. Drizzle with soy sauce and sesame oil, and toss to combine.

8. Serve chicken and vegetable stir-fry over cooked brown rice.

Servings: 2 **Nutritional Value (per serving):** Calories: 300, Protein: 25g, Fat: 8g, Carbohydrates: 30g **Cooking Time:** 20 minutes

Ingredients:

- 2 cups fresh spinach leaves

- 1 cup cooked quinoa

- 1/4 cup diced cucumber

- 1/4 cup diced bell peppers

- 2 tbsp crumbled feta cheese (optional)

- 1 tbsp chopped almonds or walnuts

- 2 tbsp lemon juice

- 1 tbsp olive oil

- Salt and pepper to taste

Instructions:

1. In a large bowl, combine fresh spinach leaves, cooked quinoa, diced cucumber, diced bell peppers, crumbled feta cheese (if using), and chopped nuts.

2. In a small bowl, whisk together lemon juice, olive oil, salt, and pepper to make the vinaigrette.

3. Drizzle the lemon vinaigrette over the salad and toss to coat evenly.

4. Serve immediately.

Servings: 2 **Nutritional Value (per serving):** Calories: 250, Protein: 10g, Fat: 12g, Carbohydrates: 30g **Preparation Time:** 15 minutes

7. Tuna Salad Lettuce Wraps

Ingredients:

- 1 can tuna, drained

- 1/4 cup diced celery

- 1/4 cup diced red onion

- 1/4 cup diced bell peppers

- 2 tbsp Greek yogurt (low-fat)

- 1 tsp Dijon mustard

- Salt and pepper to taste

- Lettuce leaves for wrapping

Instructions:

1. In a bowl, mix together drained tuna, diced celery, diced red onion, diced bell peppers, Greek yogurt, Dijon mustard, salt, and pepper.

2. Spoon the tuna salad mixture onto lettuce leaves.

3. Wrap the lettuce leaves around the tuna salad mixture.

4. Serve immediately.

Servings: 2 **Nutritional Value (per serving):** Calories: 200, Protein: 20g, Fat: 5g, Carbohydrates: 10g **Preparation Time:** 10 minutes

8. Vegetable and Lentil Curry

Ingredients:

- 1 cup cooked lentils

- 2 cups mixed vegetables (such as carrots, potatoes, peas)

- 1 onion, finely chopped

- 2 cloves garlic, minced

- 1 tbsp curry powder

- 1/2 cup coconut milk (unsweetened)

- 1 tbsp olive oil

- Salt and pepper to taste

- Fresh cilantro for garnish

Instructions:

1. Heat olive oil in a large pot over medium heat.

2. Add chopped onion and minced garlic, and cook until softened.

3. Stir in curry powder and cook for another minute.

4. Add mixed vegetables and cooked lentils to the pot.

5. Pour in coconut milk and stir to combine.

6. Simmer for 15-20 minutes or until vegetables are tender.

7. Season with salt and pepper to taste.

8. Garnish with fresh cilantro and serve hot with cooked brown rice or quinoa.

Servings: 4 **Nutritional Value (per serving):** Calories: 250, Protein: 12g, Fat: 8g, Carbohydrates: 30g **Cooking Time:** 30 minutes

Ingredients:

- 1 small eggplant, diced
- 1 can chickpeas, drained and rinsed
- 1/4 cup diced tomatoes
- 1/4 cup diced cucumber
- 1/4 cup diced red onion
- 2 tbsp chopped parsley
- 1 tbsp olive oil
- 1 tbsp lemon juice
- Salt and pepper to taste

Instructions:

1. Preheat the oven to 400°F (200°C).
2. Spread diced eggplant on a baking sheet and drizzle with olive oil.
3. Roast in the oven for 20-25 minutes or until golden brown and tender.
4. In a large bowl, combine roasted eggplant, chickpeas, diced tomatoes, diced cucumber, diced red onion, chopped parsley, olive oil, lemon juice, salt, and pepper.

5. Toss to combine and adjust seasoning if needed.

6. Serve chilled or at room temperature.

Servings: 2 **Nutritional Value (per serving):** Calories: 300, Protein: 10g, Fat: 10g, Carbohydrates: 40g **Cooking Time:** 25 minutes

10. Shrimp and Vegetable Stir-Fry

Ingredients:

- 8 oz shrimp, peeled and deveined

- 2 cups mixed vegetables (such as broccoli, snap peas, bell peppers)

- 2 cloves garlic, minced

- 1 tbsp low-sodium soy sauce

- 1 tsp sesame oil

- 1 tsp olive oil

- Cooked brown rice for serving

Instructions:

1. Heat olive oil in a large skillet or wok over medium-high heat.

2. Add minced garlic and stir-fry for 30 seconds.

3. Add shrimp to the skillet and cook until pink and opaque.

4. Remove shrimp from the skillet and set aside.

5. In the same skillet, add mixed vegetables and stir-fry until tender-crisp.

6. Return cooked shrimp to the skillet.

7. Drizzle with soy sauce and sesame oil, and toss to combine.

8. Serve shrimp and vegetable stir-fry over cooked brown rice.

Servings: 2 **Nutritional Value (per serving):** Calories: 250, Protein: 20g, Fat: 8g, Carbohydrates: 25g **Cooking Time:** 15 minutes

These osteoarthritis-friendly lunch recipes are not only delicious but also packed with nutrients to support joint health and overall well-being. Enjoy these satisfying meals while managing osteoarthritis symptoms and promoting optimal health.

Delicious osteoarthritis-friendly dinner recipes:

1. Baked Lemon Herb Chicken

Ingredients:

- 2 boneless, skinless chicken breasts
- 1 lemon, sliced
- 2 cloves garlic, minced
- 1 tbsp olive oil
- 1 tsp dried thyme
- 1 tsp dried rosemary
- Salt and pepper to taste

Instructions:

1. Preheat the oven to 375°F (190°C).
2. Place the chicken breasts in a baking dish.
3. Drizzle olive oil over the chicken breasts and rub with minced garlic, dried thyme, dried rosemary, salt, and pepper.
4. Arrange lemon slices on top of the chicken breasts.

5. Bake for 25-30 minutes or until the chicken is cooked through and juices run clear.

6. Serve hot with steamed vegetables or a side salad.

Servings: 2 **Nutritional Value (per serving):** Calories: 250, Protein: 30g, Fat: 10g, Carbohydrates: 5g **Cooking Time:** 30 minutes

2. Spaghetti Squash with Turkey Bolognese

Ingredients:

- 1 medium spaghetti squash

- 1 lb ground turkey

- 1 can diced tomatoes

- 1 onion, diced

- 2 cloves garlic, minced

- 1 tsp olive oil

- 1 tsp dried oregano

- 1 tsp dried basil

- Salt and pepper to taste

Instructions:

1. Preheat the oven to 400°F (200°C).

2. Cut the spaghetti squash in half lengthwise and scoop out the seeds.

3. Place the squash halves cut side down on a baking sheet and bake for 30-40 minutes or until tender.

4. Meanwhile, heat olive oil in a skillet over medium heat.

5. Add diced onions and minced garlic, and cook until softened.

6. Add ground turkey to the skillet and cook until browned.

7. Stir in diced tomatoes, dried oregano, dried basil, salt, and pepper.

8. Simmer for 15-20 minutes.

9. Once the spaghetti squash is cooked, use a fork to scrape the flesh into strands.

10. Serve the turkey bolognese over the spaghetti squash strands.

Servings: 4 **Nutritional Value (per serving):** Calories: 300, Protein: 25g, Fat: 10g, Carbohydrates: 30g **Cooking Time:** 60 minutes

3. Baked Salmon with Roasted Vegetables

Ingredients:

- 2 salmon fillets

- 2 cups mixed vegetables (such as carrots, zucchini, bell peppers)

- 2 tbsp olive oil

- 1 tsp dried dill

- 1 tsp garlic powder

- Salt and pepper to taste

Instructions:

1. Preheat the oven to 400°F (200°C).

2. Place the salmon fillets on a baking sheet lined with parchment paper.

3. Drizzle olive oil over the salmon fillets and sprinkle with dried dill, garlic powder, salt, and pepper.

4. In a separate baking dish, toss mixed vegetables with olive oil, salt, and pepper.

5. Arrange the vegetables around the salmon fillets on the baking sheet.

6. Bake for 15-20 minutes or until the salmon is cooked through and the vegetables are tender.

7. Serve hot.

Servings: 2 **Nutritional Value (per serving):** Calories: 300, Protein: 25g, Fat: 15g, Carbohydrates: 15g **Cooking Time:** 20 minutes

4. Cauliflower Fried Rice with Shrimp

Ingredients:

- 1 small head cauliflower, grated
- 8 oz shrimp, peeled and deveined
- 1 cup mixed vegetables (such as peas, carrots, corn)
- 2 eggs, beaten
- 2 cloves garlic, minced
- 2 tbsp low-sodium soy sauce
- 1 tbsp sesame oil
- 1 tsp olive oil
- Green onions for garnish (optional)

Instructions:

1. Heat olive oil in a large skillet or wok over medium heat.

2. Add minced garlic and stir-fry for 30 seconds.

3. Add shrimp to the skillet and cook until pink and opaque.

4. Remove shrimp from the skillet and set aside.

5. In the same skillet, add beaten eggs and scramble until cooked through.

6. Stir in grated cauliflower and mixed vegetables.

7. Cook until vegetables are tender-crisp.

8. Return cooked shrimp to the skillet.

9. Drizzle with soy sauce and sesame oil, and toss to combine.

10. Garnish with chopped green onions if desired.

11. Serve hot.

Servings: 2 **Nutritional Value (per serving):** Calories: 250, Protein: 20g, Fat: 10g, Carbohydrates: 20g **Cooking Time:** 20 minutes

Ingredients:

- 2 cod fillets
- 2 cloves garlic, minced
- 1 lemon, juiced and zested
- 1 tbsp olive oil
- 1 tsp dried parsley
- 1 tsp dried thyme
- Salt and pepper to taste

Instructions:

1. Preheat the oven to 375°F (190°C).
2. Place the cod fillets in a baking dish.
3. In a small bowl, mix together minced garlic, lemon juice, lemon zest, olive oil, dried parsley, dried thyme, salt, and pepper.
4. Pour the lemon garlic herb mixture over the cod fillets.
5. Bake for 15-20 minutes or until the cod is opaque and flakes easily with a fork.
6. Serve hot with steamed vegetables or a side salad.

Servings: 2 **Nutritional Value (per serving):** Calories: 200, Protein: 25g, Fat: 8g, Carbohydrates: 5g **Cooking Time:** 20 minutes

6. Turkey and Vegetable Stir-Fry

Ingredients:

- 1 lb ground turkey

- 2 cups mixed vegetables (such as broccoli, snap peas, bell peppers)

- 2 cloves garlic, minced

- 2 tbsp low-sodium soy sauce

- 1 tsp sesame oil

- 1 tsp olive oil

- Cooked brown rice for serving

Instructions:

1. Heat olive oil in a large skillet or wok over medium-high heat.

2. Add minced garlic and stir-fry for 30 seconds.

3. Add ground turkey to the skillet and cook until browned.

4. Add mixed vegetables to the skillet and stir-fry until tender-crisp.

5. Drizzle with soy sauce and sesame oil, and toss to combine.

6. Serve turkey and vegetable stir-fry over cooked brown rice.

Servings: 4 **Nutritional Value (per serving):** Calories: 250, Protein: 20g, Fat: 10g, Carbohydrates: 20g **Cooking Time:** 20 minutes

7. Lemon Herb Roasted Chicken and Vegetables

Ingredients:

- 2 bone-in, skin-on chicken thighs

- 1 cup mixed vegetables (such as carrots, potatoes, onions)

- 1 lemon, sliced

- 2 cloves garlic, minced

- 1 tbsp olive oil

- 1 tsp dried thyme

- 1 tsp dried rosemary

- Salt and pepper to taste

Instructions:

1. Preheat the oven to 400°F (200°C).

2. Place the chicken thighs and mixed vegetables in a baking dish.

3. Drizzle olive oil over the chicken and vegetables.

4. Rub minced garlic, dried thyme, dried rosemary, salt, and pepper onto the chicken thighs.

5. Arrange lemon slices on top of the chicken thighs.

6. Bake for 35-40 minutes or until the chicken is cooked through and the vegetables are tender.

7. Serve hot.

Servings: 2 **Nutritional Value (per serving):** Calories: 300, Protein: 25g, Fat: 15g, Carbohydrates: 15g **Cooking Time:** 40 minutes

Ingredients:

- 1 large eggplant, sliced into rounds
- 1 cup marinara sauce (low-sodium)
- 1/2 cup shredded low-fat mozzarella cheese
- 1/4 cup grated Parmesan cheese
- 1/4 cup whole wheat breadcrumbs
- 1 egg, beaten
- 1 tsp olive oil
- Fresh basil for garnish

Instructions:

1. Preheat the oven to 375°F (190°C).

2. Dip eggplant slices in beaten egg, then coat with breadcrumbs.

3. Place breaded eggplant slices on a baking sheet lined with parchment paper.

4. Bake for 15-20 minutes or until golden brown and tender.

5. In a baking dish, spread a thin layer of marinara sauce.

6. Arrange half of the baked eggplant slices on top of the marinara sauce.

7. Top with half of the shredded mozzarella cheese and grated Parmesan cheese.

8. Repeat layers with remaining ingredients.

9. Drizzle olive oil over the top layer of cheese.

10. Bake for 20-25 minutes or until the cheese is melted and bubbly.

11. Garnish with fresh basil before serving.

Servings: 2 **Nutritional Value (per serving):** Calories: 300, Protein: 15g, Fat: 10g, Carbohydrates: 30g **Cooking Time:** 45 minutes

These osteoarthritis-friendly dinner recipes are not only delicious but also packed with nutrients to support joint health and overall well-being. Enjoy these satisfying meals while managing osteoarthritis symptoms and promoting optimal health.

Delicious osteoarthritis-friendly juice and smoothie recipes:

1. Green Goddess Juice

Ingredients:

- 2 cups spinach leaves
- 1 cucumber, peeled and chopped
- 1 green apple, cored and chopped
- 1 stalk celery, chopped
- 1 inch piece of ginger, peeled
- 1 lemon, juiced
- 1 cup water or coconut water
- Ice cubes (optional)

Instructions:

1. Place all ingredients in a blender.
2. Blend until smooth.
3. If desired, strain the juice through a fine mesh sieve to remove pulp.
4. Serve immediately over ice cubes.

Servings: 2 **Nutritional Value (per serving):** Calories: 50, Protein: 2g, Fat: 0g, Carbohydrates: 12g **Preparation Time:** 5 minutes

2. Tropical Turmeric Smoothie

Ingredients:

- 1 cup frozen pineapple chunks
- 1/2 cup frozen mango chunks
- 1 banana
- 1 tsp turmeric powder
- 1/2 tsp ground cinnamon
- 1 cup unsweetened almond milk
- Ice cubes (optional)

Instructions:

1. Place all ingredients in a blender.
2. Blend until smooth.
3. Add ice cubes if desired for a colder smoothie.
4. Serve immediately.

Servings: 2 **Nutritional Value (per serving):** Calories: 150, Protein: 2g, Fat: 1g, Carbohydrates: 35g **Preparation Time:** 5 minutes

Ingredients:

- 1 cup mixed berries (such as strawberries, blueberries, raspberries)

- 1/2 banana

- 1/2 cup plain Greek yogurt (low-fat)

- 1/2 cup unsweetened almond milk

- 1 tbsp chia seeds

- Ice cubes (optional)

Instructions:

1. Place all ingredients in a blender.

2. Blend until smooth.

3. Add ice cubes if desired for a colder smoothie.

4. Serve immediately.

Servings: 1 **Nutritional Value (per serving):** Calories: 200, Protein: 10g, Fat: 5g, Carbohydrates: 30g **Preparation Time:** 5 minutes

Ingredients:

- 4 carrots, peeled and chopped

- 1 inch piece of ginger, peeled

- 1 apple, cored and chopped

- 1 lemon, juiced

- 1 cup water or coconut water

- Ice cubes (optional)

Instructions:

1. Place all ingredients in a blender.

2. Blend until smooth.

3. If desired, strain the juice through a fine mesh sieve to remove pulp.

4. Serve immediately over ice cubes.

Servings: 2 **Nutritional Value (per serving):** Calories: 60, Protein: 1g, Fat: 0g, Carbohydrates: 15g **Preparation Time:** 5 minutes

Ingredients:

- 1/2 ripe avocado
- 1 cup spinach leaves
- 1/2 banana
- 1/2 cup unsweetened almond milk
- 1 tbsp honey or maple syrup (optional)
- Ice cubes (optional)

Instructions:

1. Place all ingredients in a blender.
2. Blend until smooth.
3. Add honey or maple syrup if desired for sweetness.
4. Add ice cubes if desired for a colder smoothie.
5. Serve immediately.

Servings: 1 **Nutritional Value (per serving):** Calories: 200, Protein: 5g, Fat: 10g, Carbohydrates: 25g **Preparation Time:** 5 minutes

Ingredients:

- 2 cups chopped pineapple
- 1 inch piece of ginger, peeled
- 1 tsp turmeric powder
- 1 lemon, juiced
- 1 cup water or coconut water
- Ice cubes (optional)

Instructions:

1. Place all ingredients in a blender.
2. Blend until smooth.
3. If desired, strain the juice through a fine mesh sieve to remove pulp.
4. Serve immediately over ice cubes.

Servings: 2 **Nutritional Value (per serving):** Calories: 100, Protein: 1g, Fat: 0g, Carbohydrates: 25g **Preparation Time:** 5 minutes

Ingredients:

- 1/2 cup frozen blueberries
- 1/2 banana
- 2 tbsp almond butter
- 1 cup unsweetened almond milk
- 1 tbsp chia seeds
- Ice cubes (optional)

Instructions:

1. Place all ingredients in a blender.
2. Blend until smooth.
3. Add ice cubes if desired for a colder smoothie.
4. Serve immediately.

Servings: 1 **Nutritional Value (per serving):** Calories: 300, Protein: 8g, Fat: 15g, Carbohydrates: 35g **Preparation Time:** 5 minutes

Ingredients:

- 1 cup chopped kale leaves
- 1 cup chopped pineapple
- 1/2 banana
- 1/2 cup unsweetened coconut water
- 1 tbsp lemon juice
- Ice cubes (optional)

Instructions:

1. Place all ingredients in a blender.
2. Blend until smooth.
3. Add ice cubes if desired for a colder smoothie.
4. Serve immediately.

Servings: 1 **Nutritional Value (per serving):** Calories: 150, Protein: 3g, Fat: 1g, Carbohydrates: 35g **Preparation Time:** 5 minutes

Ingredients:

- 1 cup frozen mango chunks
- 1/2 banana
- 1 tsp turmeric powder
- 1/2 tsp ground cinnamon
- 1 cup unsweetened almond milk
- Ice cubes (optional)

Instructions:

1. Place all ingredients in a blender.
2. Blend until smooth.
3. Add ice cubes if desired for a colder smoothie.
4. Serve immediately.

Servings: 1 **Nutritional Value (per serving):** Calories: 200, Protein: 3g, Fat: 2g, Carbohydrates: 45g **Preparation Time:** 5 minutes

10. Beet Berry Smoothie

Ingredients:

- 1/2 cup cooked beets, chopped
- 1/2 cup mixed berries (such as strawberries, raspberries, blueberries)
- 1/2 banana
- 1/2 cup unsweetened almond milk
- 1 tbsp honey or maple syrup (optional)
- Ice cubes (optional)

Instructions:

1. Place all ingredients in a blender.
2. Blend until smooth.
3. Add honey or maple syrup if desired for sweetness.
4. Add ice cubes if desired for a colder smoothie.
5. Serve immediately.

Servings: 1 Nutritional Value (per serving): Calories: 150, Protein: 3g, Fat: 1g, Carbohydrates: 35g **Preparation Time:** 5 minutes

These osteoarthritis-friendly juice and smoothie recipes are not only delicious but also packed with nutrients to support joint health and overall well-being. Enjoy these refreshing beverages as part of your daily routine to manage osteoarthritis symptoms and promote optimal health.

CONCLUSION:

The Osteoarthritis Diet Cookbook offers a comprehensive guide to managing osteoarthritis symptoms through delicious and nutritious recipes. By incorporating calcium-rich, vitamin D-rich, low-sugar, low-carb, and low-fat ingredients, each recipe is carefully crafted to support joint health and overall well-being. From hearty breakfasts to satisfying lunches and comforting dinners, this cookbook provides a wide variety of options to suit every taste preference.

Through the power of nutrition, you can take control of your osteoarthritis journey and experience relief from joint pain and inflammation. By fueling the body with nutrient-dense foods, you can enhance bone health, improve mobility, and enjoy a better quality of life.

Remember, adopting an osteoarthritis-friendly diet is not just about managing symptoms—it's about embracing a lifestyle that prioritizes health and vitality. By nourishing your body with wholesome ingredients and flavorful meals, you're not only treating your osteoarthritis but also investing in your long-term well-being.

So, why wait? Take the first step towards a healthier, happier life today by incorporating the recipes from this Cookbook into your daily routine. Let food be thy medicine, and embark on a journey towards optimal health and vitality. Your joints will thank you, and you'll discover a renewed sense of vitality and wellness that comes from nourishing your body from the inside out.

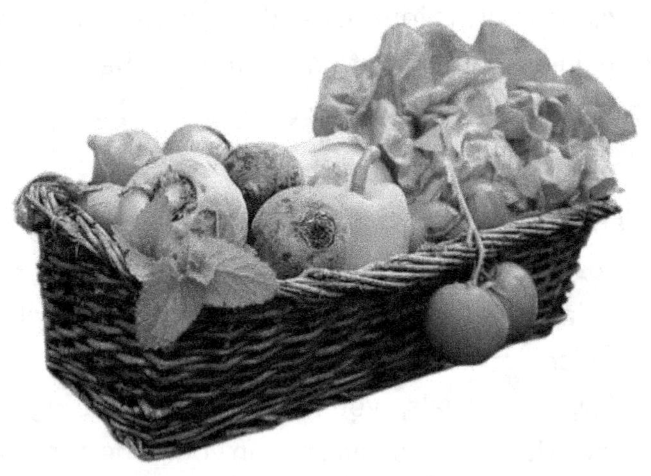

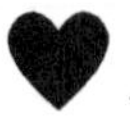 

THANK YOU FOR READING

Thank you for joining us on our journey towards better joint health and well-being. If you've found this cookbook to be a valuable resource in your quest to manage osteoarthritis, I would greatly appreciate it if you could take a moment to share your thoughts through a rating or review. Your feedback fuels my passion for providing top-notch recipes and guidance.

I understand that managing osteoarthritis can be daunting, so I am here to support you every step of the way. If any part of this cookbook leaves you with questions or uncertainties, please don't hesitate to reach out to me at drmarydcook@gmail.com . I am committed to helping you thrive and inspire others to take charge of their joint health.

Together, let's inspire others to take charge of their joint health and embrace a lifestyle of wellness. Thank you again for choosing to embark on this transformative path with me.

Here's to your continued health, vitality, and happiness!

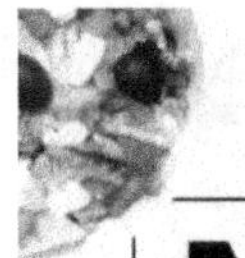

MEAL
PLANNER

DATE:

	BREAKFAST	LUNCH	DINNER	SHOPPING LIST
MON				
TUES				
WED				
THURS				
FRI				
SAT				
SUN				

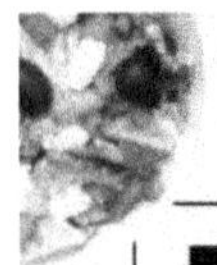

MEAL PLANNER

DATE: ___________

	BREAKFAST	LUNCH	DINNER	SHOPPING LIST
MON				
TUES				
WED				
THURS				
FRI				
SAT				
SUN				

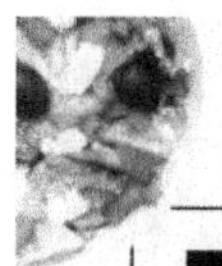
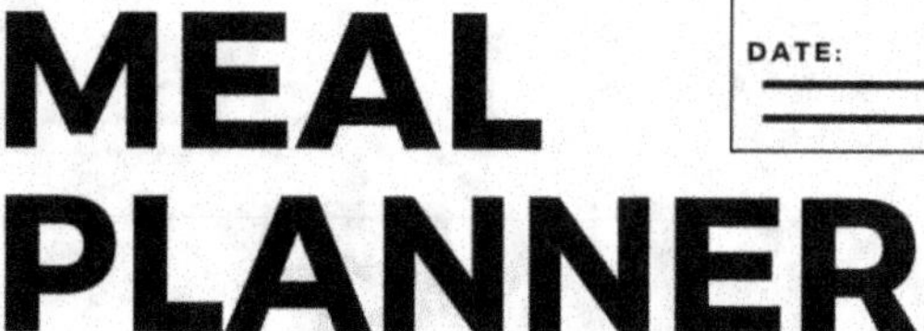

MEAL PLANNER

DATE: _______________

	BREAKFAST	LUNCH	DINNER	SHOPPING LIST
MON				
TUES				
WED				
THURS				
FRI				
SAT				
SUN				

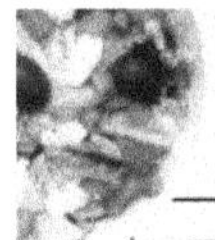

MEAL PLANNER

DATE:

	BREAKFAST	LUNCH	DINNER	SHOPPING LIST
MON				
TUES				
WED				
THURS				
FRI				
SAT				
SUN				

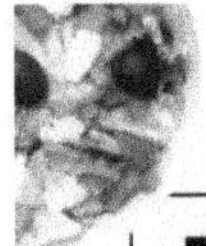
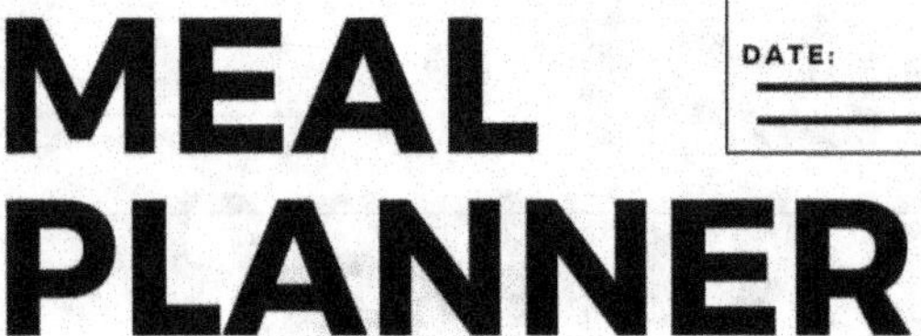

MEAL
PLANNER

DATE:

	BREAKFAST	LUNCH	DINNER	SHOPPING LIST
MON				
TUES				
WED				
THURS				
FRI				
SAT				
SUN				

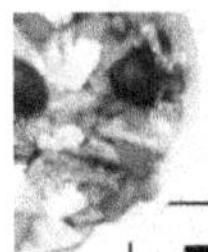
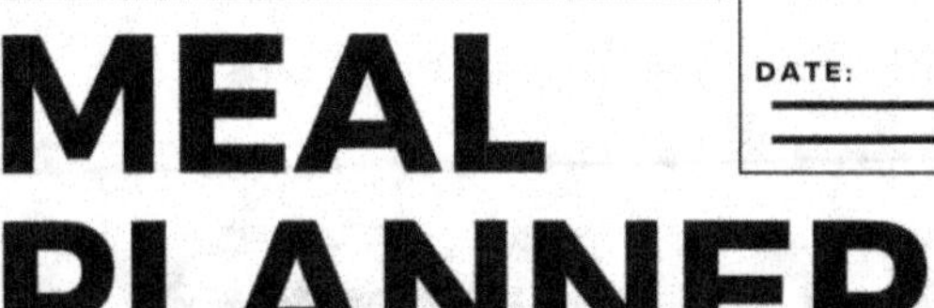

MEAL PLANNER

DATE:

	BREAKFAST	LUNCH	DINNER	SHOPPING LIST
MON				
TUES				
WED				
THURS				
FRI				
SAT				
SUN				

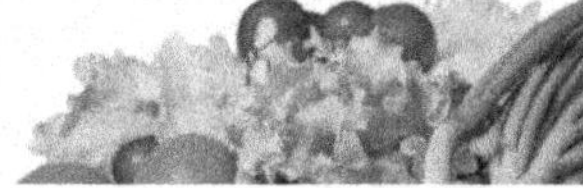

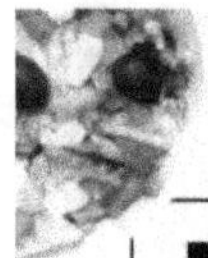

MEAL PLANNER

DATE: ___________

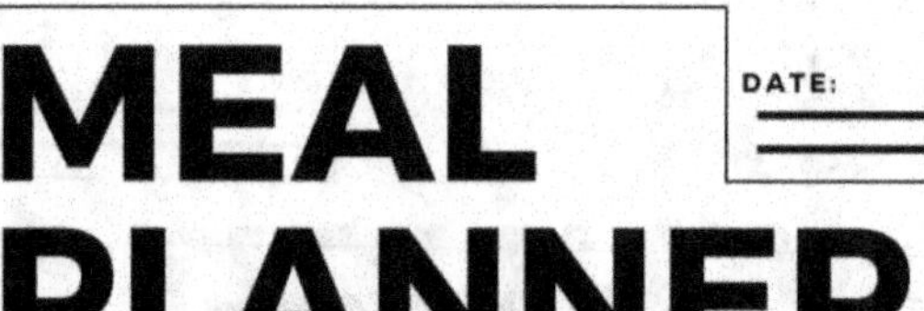

	BREAKFAST	LUNCH	DINNER	SHOPPING LIST
MON				
TUES				
WED				
THURS				
FRI				
SAT				
SUN				

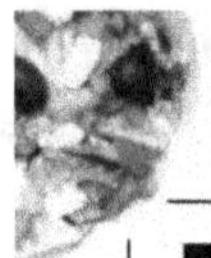

MEAL PLANNER

DATE:

	BREAKFAST	LUNCH	DINNER	SHOPPING LIST
MON				
TUES				
WED				
THURS				
FRI				
SAT				
SUN				

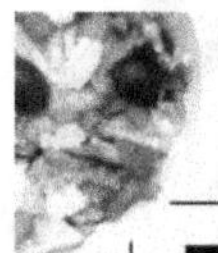

MEAL PLANNER

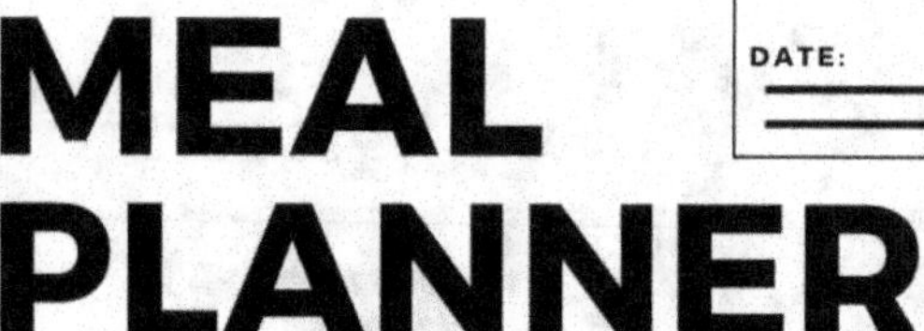

DATE: ___________

	BREAKFAST	LUNCH	DINNER	SHOPPING LIST
MON				
TUES				
WED				
THURS				
FRI				
SAT				
SUN				

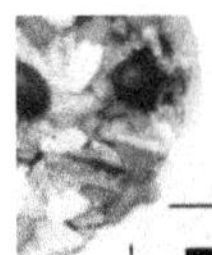

MEAL PLANNER

DATE:

	BREAKFAST	LUNCH	DINNER	SHOPPING LIST
MON				
TUES				
WED				
THURS				
FRI				
SAT				
SUN				

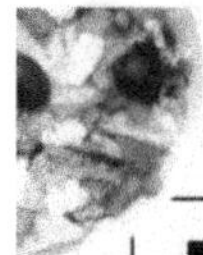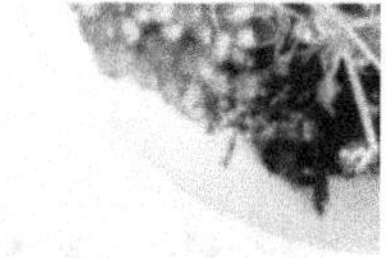

MEAL
PLANNER

DATE:

	BREAKFAST	LUNCH	DINNER	SHOPPING LIST
MON				
TUES				
WED				
THURS				
FRI				
SAT				
SUN				

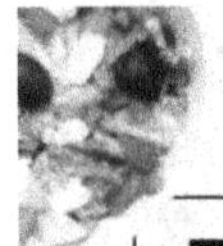
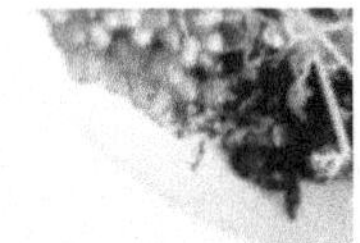

MEAL
PLANNER

DATE:

	BREAKFAST	LUNCH	DINNER	SHOPPING LIST
MON				
TUES				
WED				
THURS				
FRI				
SAT				
SUN				

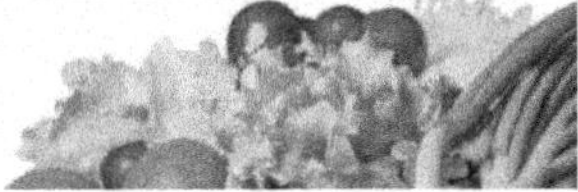

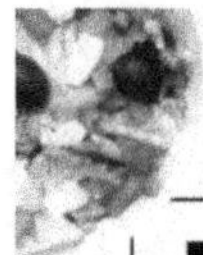
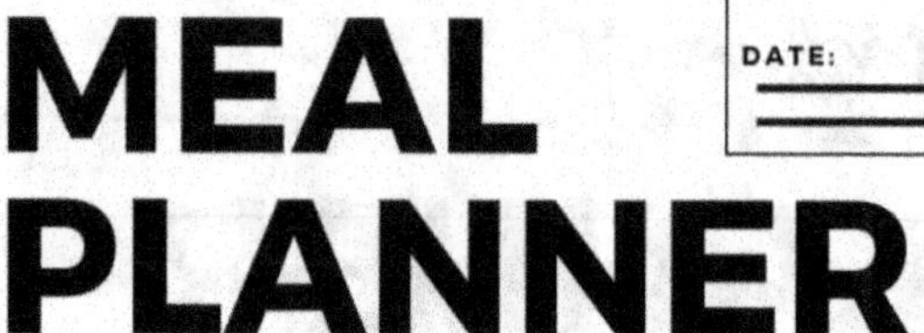

MEAL PLANNER

DATE: ___________

	BREAKFAST	LUNCH	DINNER	SHOPPING LIST
MON				
TUES				
WED				
THURS				
FRI				
SAT				
SUN				

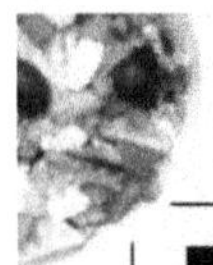
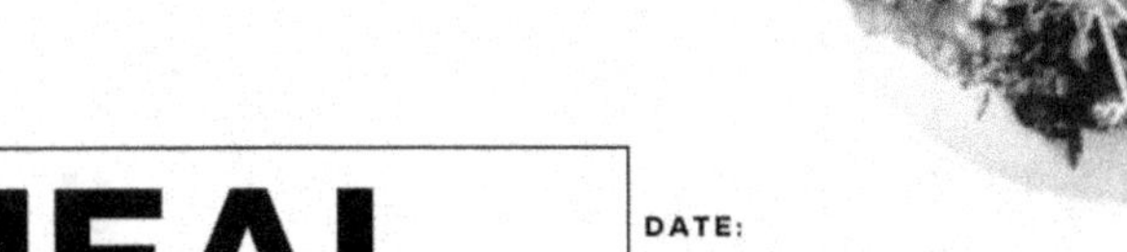

MEAL PLANNER

DATE:

	BREAKFAST	LUNCH	DINNER	SHOPPING LIST
MON				
TUES				
WED				
THURS				
FRI				
SAT				
SUN				

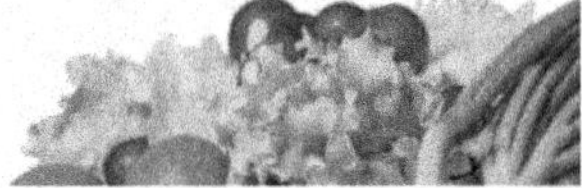